Mariane Carolina de Almeida
Eduardo J. Souza
Fabiana M. Dallacosta

Dialysis Quality

Mariane Carolina de Almeida
Eduardo J. Souza
Fabiana M. Dallacosta

Dialysis Quality

Caring for patients with Chronic Kidney Disease

ScienciaScripts

Imprint

Cover image: www.ingimage.com

This book is a translation from the original published under ISBN 978-613-9-69937-7.

Publisher:
Sciencia Scripts
is a trademark of
Dodo Books Indian Ocean Ltd. and OmniScriptum S.R.L publishing group

120 High Road, East Finchley, London, N2 9ED, United Kingdom
Str. Armeneasca 28/1, office 1, Chisinau MD-2012, Republic of Moldova, Europe
Printed at: see last page
ISBN: 978-620-8-14223-0

"The rung of a ladder is not for resting, but for supporting the foot for as long as it takes for the man to place the other foot a little higher."

(Aldous Huxley)

SUMMARY

The aim of this study was to assess the adequacy of haemodialysis in chronic patients undergoing treatment at a private clinic in the midwest of Santa Catarina. This is a cross-sectional, qualitative study. The study comprised 29 patients undergoing haemodialysis through an arteriovenous fistula. Blood samples were taken and sent to the laboratory for urea testing. It was observed that the majority of the sample had either intermediate or high recirculation rates, while the changes observed in the Urea Reduction Rate (URR) and the Kt/V equation were less significant. Gender and age did not significantly affect the increase in the levels of the changes found in the recirculation parameter. It was concluded that, in general, the treatment is being efficient and adequate and that the dialysis adequacy parameters once again proved to be important tools, since they were able to detect the efficiency and/or inefficiency of the dialysis procedure. Keywords: Haemodialysis. Arteriovenous Fistula. Adequacy.

SUMMARY

CHAPTER 1

INTRODUCTION

The choice of research topic is fundamental, according to Cabral et al (2013, p. 16) "Kidney disease is currently considered a serious public health problem, not only because of the high morbidity and mortality but also because of the low quality of life that this disease brings to these patients." Chronic renal failure (CRF) is a progressive and irreversible disease due to a major impairment of kidney function, caused by uncontrolled chronic diseases that affect the kidneys associated with risk factors such as sedentary lifestyle, smoking, excessive alcohol consumption, eating habits, stress, among others (CABRAL et al., 2013). In addition, CRF affects a large part of the population. In this pathology there is kidney damage, where the kidney is unable to carry out the normal processes of filtration, reabsorption and secretion. This is important since the body needs the kidney functions to be preserved in order to maintain homeostasis, which therefore justifies the need for haemodialysis (HD) or other forms of dialysis in this condition (WOLOSKER; KUZNIEC, 2007).

Haemodialysis is an invasive procedure in which extracorporeal circulation is carried out in the dialysis bath via a venous access (permanent or temporary). Thus, haemodialysis is characterised by a therapy which provides solute exchange by diffusion between the patient's blood and the dialysis solution through a semi-permeable membrane (capillary). In this way, the client's blood moves through the vascular access route to the capillary where it is purified through a cardiopulmonary bypass circuit, which begins and ends in the patient's circulatory system (WOLOSKER;

KUZNIEC, 2007).

Over the years, new technologies have emerged in the field of haemodialysis, among which various forms of venous access have been developed and improved. One of them, which was used in this study, is the Arteriovenous Fistula (AVF), which is characterised by a surgical procedure in which a vein is connected to an artery (KOEPE; ARAÚJO, 2008). Four to six weeks after the procedure, the vein (most commonly the cephalic vein) dilates and its wall thickens due to the pulsating action of the artery (in this case the radial artery), which makes it more durable and resistant to constant punctures (REIS et al., 2001). The needles are then inserted into the vessel in order to obtain better circulation to pass through the dialyser (KOEPE; ARAÚJO, 2008). In addition, according to the Dialysis Manual/Nephrology Service of the Getúlio Vargas Hospital (2012 p.23) "The punctures of the arterial and venous branches should be 5 cm apart, avoiding blood recirculation." Furthermore, the AVF will take time to mature, but in some situations the client needs haemodialysis as soon as possible. In these cases, temporary catheters need to be implanted, which expose the patient to possible complications (WOLOSKER; KUZNIEC, 2007).

A major advance in dialysis treatment is the quantification of haemodialysis, which has great importance for the morbidity and mortality of chronic kidney patients. Adequate dialysis is dialysis that can be verified and therefore minimises the client's morbidity and mortality. This verification refers to adequacy, which is based on uremic principles, signs and symptoms presented by the client and calculations that will measure the quality of dialysis (DRAIBE; CENDOROGLO; NADALETTO, 2000).

Thus, quantifying dialysis is the first step towards its adequacy (KDOQI, 2006).

The ultimate goal of dialysis is to reduce the levels of solutes through their clearance, in which case urea is considered a good marker because it is easily dialysed, i.e. urea concentrations decrease significantly during treatment. The rapid and intermittent drop in serum urea concentration during HD allows us to easily measure the dose found in patients (KDOQI, 2006). If the urea concentration is altered, it is an important indication that the circulation is not being effective, so the nurse, together with the team, should look for ways to make haemodialysis successful (MANUAL DE DIÁLISE/SERVIÇO DE NEFROLOGIA DO HOSPITAL GETÚLIO VARGAS, 2012).

To adjust haemodialysis, a number of equations have been standardised based on serum urea values. These include:

- Blood Recirculation, a calculation proposed by D'Avilla (DALLACOSTA; FIGUEIREDO, 2010);
- the Urea Reduction Rate (URR) equation developed by Lowrie and Lew (1991) *apud* Shinaberger (2001);
- and the Second Generation Logarithmic Formula, with the calculation of Kt/V, proposed by Daugirdas (1993) and endorsed by KDOQI (2006).

The equations mentioned above use pre- and post-dialysis urea values. The result of these calculations reflects the efficiency of dialysis, as well as representing important parameters of dialysis adequacy to be assessed by the HD nurse.

CHAPTER 2

GENERAL OBJECTIVE

The aim of this study was to assess the quality (adequacy) of haemodialysis in chronic patients dialysing at a private clinic in the midwest of Santa Catarina.

2.1 OJECTIVES

- Calculate urea recirculation.
- Calculation of URR *(urea reduction ratio).*
- Calculate Kt V.

CHAPTER 3

LITERATURE REVIEW

With each heart contraction, 1.2 litres of blood pass through the kidney per minute, and the entire blood volume of the body is filtered by the kidney 340 times a day. The kidneys are located in a retroperitoneal position in the abdomen, one on each side of the spine, and are protected by a tough fibrous capsule, the renal capsule. They are approximately 12 cm long, 6 cm wide and 2.5 cm thick, and weigh around 125 to 170 grams in men and 115 to 155 grams in women. By checking the size and weight of the kidneys, a differential diagnosis of renal failure can be made using ultrasound (MORTON, 2007). The adrenal gland is located at the apex of each kidney, and each organ *is* independent in terms of its function, blood supply and innervation (BRUNNER; SUDDARTH et al., 2009).

2.2 FUNCTIONS OF THE RENAL SYSTEM

The renal system is responsible for balancing the concentration of solutes in the extracellular fluid, removing metabolic waste products and excessive concentrations of constituents (MORTON, 2007). To understand the importance of the renal system, you need to know about its functions.

2.2.1 **Renal *clearance***

It refers to the ability of the kidneys to purify (remove) solutes from the plasma (BRUNNER; SUDDARTH et al., 2009). Renal metabolic products are purified from the blood and leave the body through urine. Of every 125 ml of glomerular filtrate formed per minute, approximately 60 ml returns to the body without urea, and the rest is excreted as urea, so 60 ml of plasma is purified. In the same way, 125 ml of plasma is cleared of creatinine, 12 ml of uric acid, 12 ml of potassium, among the other solutes cleared (MORTON, 2007).

3.1. **2Regulation**

The kidneys help regulate electrolyte concentrations (including sodium, potassium, chloride, calcium, phosphorus and magnesium) and also help regulate the pH of the blood and the body's interstitial fluid (MORTON, 2007).

3.1.3Other **functions**

The renal interstitial cells produce and secrete erythropoietin (a glycoprotein hormone that stimulates the bone marrow to produce red blood cells) and calcitriol (a hormone that increases plasma calcium concentration), hormones that are important for the body's homeostasis. In addition, the renal system activates vitamin D (important for calcium absorption) (MORTON, 2007).

3. 2ACUTE RENAL FAILURE (ARF)

It is a reversible clinical syndrome in which there is a sudden and almost complete loss of kidney function over days or hours, where the clearance of solutes is not happening efficiently, causing an increase in the plasma concentration of creatinine and urea (BRUNNER; SUDDARTH et al., 2009). The main categories of ARF are Pre-renal (hypoperfusion of the kidney); Intra-renal (impairment of renal tissue); and Post-renal (obstruction of urine flow) (DIEPENBROCK, 2005).

3. 3CHRONIC RENAL FAILURE

It results from the destruction of kidney tissue with the consequent gradual loss of kidney function. Its symptoms are silent, so that when the disease is diagnosed only 25% of the kidney is carrying out glomerular filtration. As kidney function decreases, the symptoms become more pronounced and can lead to death. Some of the causes of CRF are classified:

glomerulonephritis, chronic pyelonephritis, congenital anomalies (polycystic kidney), hypertension, obstruction, among others (ANTCZAK et al., 2005).

3.4 UREA

Urea has been used as an indicator of kidney function for many years and its concentration can be influenced by many factors. Increased production of this solute may be related to the patient's increased protein intake, and is characterised as an indication for haemodialysis, as well as Chronic Renal Failure and in the complications of Acute Renal Failure (MORTON, 2007).

During the period in which the patient is undergoing haemodialysis, urea remains an important indicator of Dialysis Adequacy, reflecting the effectiveness of dialysis, as high urea levels indicate inadequate clearance. Uremia must be corrected in order to avoid imbalance syndrome, including signs and symptoms such as headache, nausea, vomiting, confusion, convulsions, agitation, among others (MORTON, 2007). Urea is a low molecular weight toxin (molecular weight 60), so its clearance is rapid and intermittent, while high molecular weight molecules are not cleared (KDOQI, 2006).

3.5 HEMODIALYSIS

HD is a procedure used when the kidneys are no longer able to carry out their physiological activities, due to relevant clinical conditions such as ARF and CRF, which lead to loss of renal system function. In order for the body to maintain homeostasis, it needs preserved kidney function, due to the clearance of solutes, which increases patient mortality rates (WOLOSKER; KUZNIEC, 2007).

3.5.1 **HD procedure**

HD is a process in which a solution S (blood) is used and then altered by exposure to a second solution B (dialysis bath) through a semi-permeable membrane. This membrane is like a sheet full of pores. With this exposure, water molecules and low-molecular-weight solutes from the two solutions will pass through the membrane's pores; however, larger solutes (such as proteins) cannot pass through this membrane, so the quantities of high-molecular-weight solutes will remain unchanged. We call this dynamic of solute exchange Solute Transport Mechanisms that occur by diffusion and ultrafiltration (MANUAL DE DIÁLISE/SERVIÇO DE NEFROLOGIA DO HOSPITAL GETÚLIO VARGAS, 2012).

To carry out dialysis, the patient needs a venous access, which can be temporary or permanent. An example of temporary access is the Percutaneous Venous Catheter, which uses the internal jugular vein or the right or left subclavian vein. This type of access is indicated in cases of ARF or CRF in patients who do not have permanent access. An example of permanent access is the arteriovenous fistula, which is characterised as an invasive procedure where an anastomosis is made between an artery and a vein, and is therefore considered the safest and longest-lasting vascular access. The most classic access is from the cephalic vein to the radial artery (MANUAL DE DIÁLISE DA NEFROCLÍNICA, 2011). After the AVF has matured for approximately four to six weeks (REIS et al, 2001), a puncture is made in the arterial branch and another in the venous branch, which should be 5 cm apart, as shown in figures 1 and 2 (NEFROCLINIC DIALYSIS MANUAL, 2011).

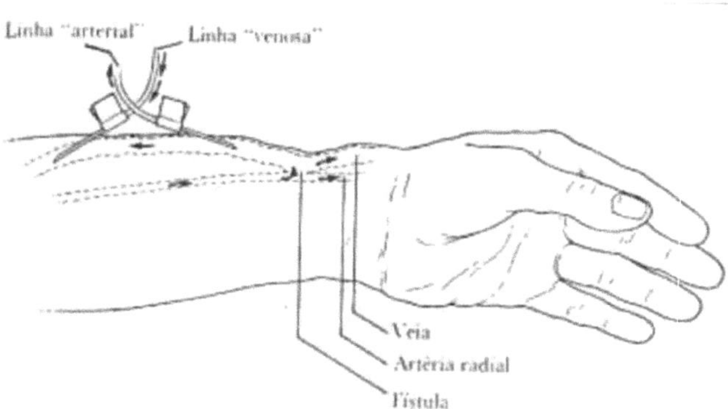

Figure 1: Representation of venous access in the arterial branch and venous branch of the arteriovenous fistula.

Source: Nefroclínica Dialysis Manual, 2011.

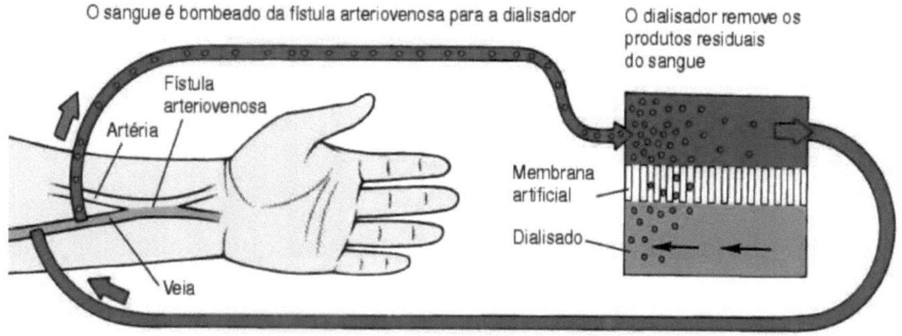

Figure 2: Diagram representing the HD procedure, showing the blood leaving the venous access, then passing through the dialyser and then returning to the client.

Source: AKISKAL et al., 2009.

3.5.2Care of **the AVF**

Nurses should advise patients and their families on how to care for the AVF. Therefore, precautions such as not checking blood pressure in the arm with the arteriovenous fistula, or not sleeping on the arm with the arteriovenous fistula, should be taken.

In addition, avoiding the administration of intravenous medication in the fistula access, exercising the arm with extension and flexion movements in order to prevent oedema, are important for the proper functioning of the HD access (MANUAL DE DIÁLISE/SERVIÇO DE NEFROLOGIA DO HOSPITAL GETÚLIO VARGAS, 2012).

Nurses must be attentive and guide their team to the first signs of AVF infection, such as oedema, erythema, the presence of exudate or fever. They should also emphasise the importance of good asepsis, using the correct puncture technique, alternating puncture sites, securing needles to avoid trauma and bleeding, applying pressure after removing the needles in order to stop the bleeding and dressings should be compressive, kept clean and dry (NEFROCLINIC DIALYSIS MANUAL, 2011).

3.5.3 **Patient monitoring**

According to Daugirdas (2008), it is important to pay attention to a few factors before and during dialysis:

- Weight: the patient's pre-dialysis weight should be compared with the last post-dialysis weight and with the dry weight to be obtained at the end of dialysis, in order to have some idea of inter-dialysis weight gain. If the patient has a large dialysis weight gain, if associated with orthopnoea or dyspnoea, they should be referred for a cardiovascular examination and their dry weight should be reassessed. Patients should also be advised to limit their water intake and try to keep their weight gain below 1.0kg per day. The symptom of thirst may indicate a high level of sodium in the dialysis solution, and complaints of muscle cramps and fatigue indicate that the target dry weight is too low.

- Blood pressure: hypertension in the pre-dialysis phase may be associated with fluid volume, but due to the renin system, many patients may experience hypertension during dialysis, even with volume withdrawal. Patients who use antihypertensive drugs are advised to discontinue use on the day of dialysis in order to prevent cases of hypotension during dialysis.

- Temperature: the temperature should be measured before dialysis, as it is a very important finding that deserves detailed investigation. It should also be measured during dialysis, but an increase of 0.5^0 is considered normal during haemodialysis.

- Access site: regardless of whether the patient has a fever or not, the access should always be assessed, always looking for signs of infection before each dialysis.

- Monitoring during the dialysis session: blood pressure and pulse are normally checked every 30 to 60 minutes. At any sign of hypotension, the patient's pressure should be checked, as it can drop to dangerous levels.

- Laboratory tests: Plasma urea nitrogen should be measured monthly due to the increased risk of mortality. Plasma albumin should be measured every 3 months as it is an important indicator of the client's nutritional status. Creatinine is also measured monthly, as it is an indicator of muscle mass and nutritional status. Creatinine and urea values should be strictly evaluated, as parallel changes in these parameters are an important factor in changing the dialysis regime. Other important tests are plasma cholesterol, potassium, phosphorus, calcium, bicarbonate, haematocrit and others.

3.6 SUITABILITY FOR DIALYSIS

To ensure that patients with Chronic Kidney Disease (CKD) treated with HD receive adequate treatment, we must use parameters that indicate the efficiency or inefficiency of the dialysis procedure (KDOQI, 2006). Thanks to the rapid intermittent drop in urea concentration (due to it being a low molecular weight toxin) (DAUGIRDAS, 2008) during HD, it is relatively easy to measure the concentration of this solute. Signs and symptoms (especially uremic symptoms) alone are not reliable indicators of dialysis adequacy, and quantification of pre- and post-dialysis urea values is necessary (KDOQI, 2006). One way of quantifying dialysis is through three different equations: Blood Recirculation, URR and Kt/V. These equations will be demonstrated below.

3.6.1 **Blood recirculation**

Blood Recirculation is an important parameter for assessing dialysis efficiency, which uses pre- and post-dialysis urea values. The calculation was proposed by D'Avilla, in which (DALLACOSTA; FIGUEIREDO, 2010):

$$\%R = (S-A) / (S-V) \times 100$$

S is the result of the laboratory examination of the blood sample taken from the arterial line, in the second phase of collection; A is the result of the laboratory examination of the blood sample from the arterial line, considered the pre-dialysis urea level; V is the result of the laboratory examination of the blood sample from the venous line, considered the post-dialysis urea level. The number 100 is the transformation into a percentage (MANUAL DE DIÁLISE/SERVIÇO DE NEFROLOGIA DO HOSPITAL GETÚLIO VARGAS, 2012).

In general, the AVF should have low recirculation under normal conditions, but some factors such as placing the puncture needles too close together can alter recirculation levels (MANUAL DE DIÁLISE/SERVIÇO DE NEFROLOGIA DO HOSPITAL GETÚLIO VARGAS, 2012). The result of this equation will be obtained as a percentage, where a value <10% is considered Low Recirculation, from 10% to 20% Intermediate Recirculation, and a value >20% is considered High Recirculation (NEFROCLINIC DIALYSIS MANUAL, 2011).

3.6.2 **URR**

Another measure of haemodialysis adequacy was used, the URR (urea reduction rate) formula developed by Lowrie and Lew (1991) *apud* Shinaberger (2001), in which:

URR= 100 (Ureapre-Ureiapós)/Ureiapré

URR *(Urea reduction rate);* Ureapre (u*rea* before haemodialysis in mg/dl); Ureaafter (urea after haemodialysis in mg/dl) (KDOQI, 2006).

As noted, the pre- and post-dialysis urea values are also used to arrive at the result, which will be given as a percentage. Direct measurement of URR has been proposed as a simpler substitute for complex equations or formal urea modelling to calculate the dialysis dose. An acceptable value is considered to be > 65% (KDOQI, 2006).

3.6.3 **Kt/V**

Another important formula for dialysis adequacy is the Second Generation Logarithmic Formula (fractional clearance of urea), which uses Kt/V parameters (where K is the clearance of urea, t is the dialysis time and V is the volume of distribution). In this formula some factors are used such as the decrease in serum urea during dialysis; the reduction in the volume of water in the body; and the generation of urea during treatment.

The values considered normal for Kt/V should be >1.2 (KDOQI, 2006). The equation was proposed by Daugirdas (1993) and endorsed by KDOQI (2006) and is summarised as follows:

Kt/V= -In (R - 0.008 . t) + (4- 3.5 . R).UF/weight

In is the natural logarithm; R is the post/pre dialysis urea concentration ratio; t is the duration of haemodialysis in hours and UF *is* the ultrafiltration in litres and weight in kg. To calculate Kt/V, dialysis time and volume must be determined precisely (KDOQI, 2006).

CHAPTER 4

METHODOLOGY

4.1 TYPE OF STUDY

Cross-sectional, quantitative study.

4.2 POPULATION

Patients undergoing haemodialysis at a private clinic in the Midwest of Santa Catarina were used in this study. The data was collected between June and August 2014.

4.3 DATA COLLECTION

First of all, the coordinator of the haemodialysis clinic personally asked for permission to carry out the research.

According to the venous access recirculation routine, after 30 minutes from the start of haemodialysis the Ultra-filtration (UF) was switched off, maintaining a normal blood flow. The first sample was taken from the arterial line (3 ml, sample A), the second from the venous line (3 ml, sample V). In the second phase of collection, the flow was reduced to 100 ml/min, 15 seconds were waited and the blood pump was switched off. Subsequently, the arterial line was clamped immediately after the collection point and a blood sample was taken from the arterial line (3ml, sample S). After all the samples had been collected, the clamp was opened and the blood pump was switched on, returning to normal blood flow, and the UF was reactivated (MANUAL DE DIÁLISE/SERVIÇO DE NEFROLOGIA

DO HOSPITAL GETÚLIO VARGAS, 2012).

The samples were then sent for laboratory testing to determine urea levels. The formula proposed by D'Avilla was used to calculate recirculation (DALLACOSTA; FIGUEIREDO, 2010):

$$\%R= (S-A) / (S-V) X 100$$

We also used another measure of haemodialysis adequacy developed by Lowrie and Lew (1991) *apud* Shinaberger (2001), in which:

URR= 100 (Ureapre-Ureiapós)/Ureiapré

URR *{Urea reduction rate),* Ureapre (urea before haemodialysis in mg/dl), Ureaafter (*urea* after haemodialysis in mg/dl). In this case, 1 ml of pre-hemodialysis serum and 1 ml of post-hemodialysis serum were used (KDOQI, 2006).

Another measure of adequacy was used, the calculation of Kt/V (Total fractional urea clearance), the result of adding the Kt/V of haemodialysis and the patient's renal Kt/V known as the Second Generation Logarithmic Formula (fractional urea *clearance*), in which K is the clearance of urea, t is the dialysis time and V is the volume of distribution. In this case we needed data such as pre- and post-dialysis urea, dialysis time in hours, how many litres of ultrafiltration (UF), post-dialysis weight. The equation by Daugirdas (1993) endorsed by KDOQI (2006) is summarised as follows:

$$Kt/V= -In (R - 0.008 . t) + (4- 3.5 . R).UF/weight$$

In is the natural logarithm; R is the post/pre dialysis urea concentration ratio; t is the duration of haemodialysis in hours and UF is the ultrafiltration in litres and weight in kg (KDOQI, 2006). The Dialysis Efficiency (Kt/V)

Calculator programme was used to calculate Kt/V and confirm the URR results.

4.4 INCLUSION CRITERIA

- Over 18 years of age;
- Have been on haemodialysis for at least six months prior to data collection;

-Use the arteriovenous fistula as dialysis access.

4.5 EXCLUSION CRITERIA

- Not agreeing to take part in the study;
- Use catheter as dialysis access.

4.6 ETHICAL ASPECTS

All patients were informed of the collection procedure and their authorisation was requested in advance by means of an Informed Consent Form. Due to the fact that the research involved human beings, it was previously submitted for analysis by the ethics committee and approved by opinion 113.

4.7 STATISTICAL ANALYSIS

Where appropriate, Student's t-test was used to compare two independent groups. The value adopted for statistical significance was £><0.05. No statistical analysis was carried out on the data from patients who had alterations in the URR and Kt/V parameters, since only a very small number of patients had alterations in these parameters.

The graphs were drawn up using *GraphPad Prism* 5.0® software and Microsoft Excel 2010. The data was analysed using the STATISTICA 7 statistical program.

CHAPTER 5

RESULTS

The sample population used in this study consisted of 29 patients who had been undergoing haemodialysis at a private clinic in the Midwest of Santa Catarina for a minimum treatment period of six months prior to data collection.

The age of the patients ranged from 29 to 81 years, with an average of 57.31 years and a Standard Deviation (SD) of 14.32. In addition, with regard to the number of clients undergoing haemodialysis treatment, there was a predominance of males - 18 clients (62%) - compared to females - 11 clients (38%) (data not shown).

5.1 RECIRCULATION

With regard to serum urea recirculation, 12 patients (42%) had low recirculation (<10%), 12 patients (41%) had intermediate recirculation (10% to 20%) and five patients (17%) had high recirculation (>20%) (Graph 1). The mean recirculation was 13.22 with a SD of 9.93.

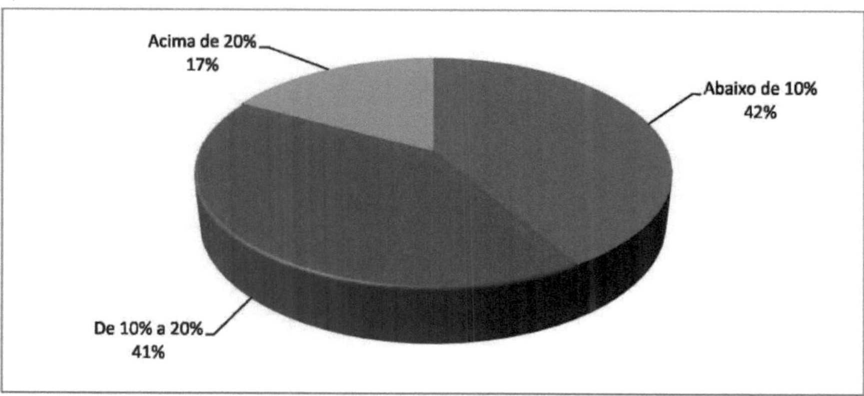

Graph 1: Distribution profile of patients undergoing haemodialysis at a private clinic in the

Midwest according to the recirculation rate criterion.
Source: the author.

The data above represents the distribution of the total number of 29 patients (n= 29), classified according to the rate of recirculation according to criteria that indicate dialysis efficiency: low recirculation (<10%), intermediate recirculation (10% to 20%) and high recirculation (>20%). All the patients had previously been randomly selected because they had an arteriovenous fistula. It is important to note that 17% of the patients had a high recirculation rate, which is considered to be higher than that accepted as indicative of efficiency (>20%) for the dialysis procedure.

5.2 URR

With regard to the urea reduction rate (URR), it was observed that seven patients (24%) had an URR below 65%, while 22 patients had an URR > 65% (Graph 2). It is important to remember that the urea reduction rate must be > 65% to express dialysis efficiency. The average URR was 69.82 with a SD of 7.32.

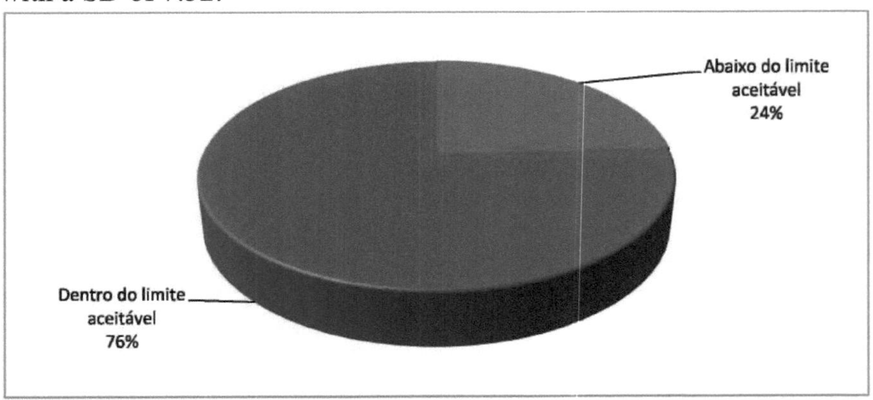

Graph 2: Distribution profile of patients undergoing haemodialysis at a private clinic in the Midwest according to the circulating urea reduction rate (URR) criterion.
Source: the author.

The data above represents the distribution of the total number of 29 patients (n= 29), classified according to their URR according to a criterion indicating dialysis efficiency (value > 65%). All the patients had previously been randomly selected because they had an arteriovenous fistula. It is important to note that when this parameter is assessed, the majority of the samples analysed (76%) have URR values that are within those established as indicative of efficiency (> 65%) for the dialysis procedure.

5. 3Kt/V

With regard to Kt/V, only 3 patients (10%) had a value below 1.2, while 26 patients (90%) had Kt/V values > 1.2, indicating that the vast majority of patients were within the range considered normal for this parameter (Graph 3). The general average (of the 29 patients) for KT/V was 1.61 and SD 0.38.

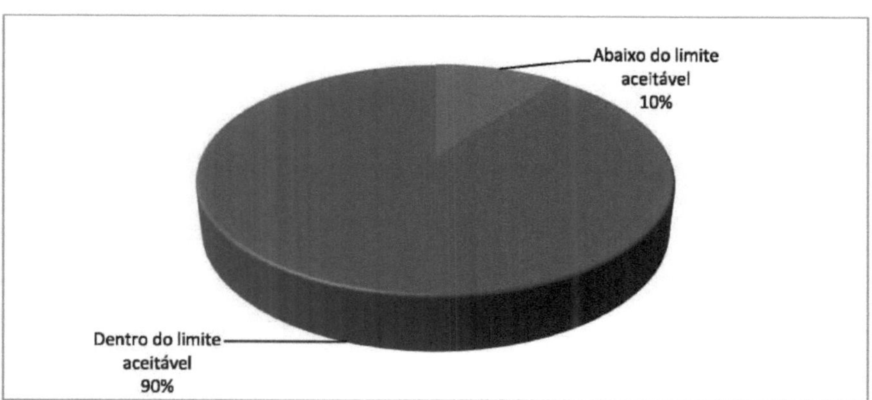

Graph 3: Distribution profile of patients undergoing haemodialysis at a private clinic in the Midwest according to the Kt/V index criterion presented.

Source: the author.

The data represents the distribution of the total number of 29 patients (n= 29), classified according to the Kt/V value presented according to the following criteria indicative of dialysis efficiency (value > 1.2). All the patients were previously randomly selected because they had an arteriovenous fistula. It is important to note that, when assessing this parameter, the majority of the samples analysed (90%) had Kt/V values that were within those established as indicative of dialysis efficiency.

5.4 INFLUENCE OF GENDER ON DIALYSIS PARAMETERS

The gender factor was analysed in detail in relation to the changes observed in the dialysis adequacy parameters stipulated in this study (Graph 4):

- Among the urea recirculation rates characterising an intermediate or high alteration, nine male patients were found compared to eight female patients who also presented such alterations.

- In the urea reduction rate, six male patients and only one female patient had a rate of less than 65%.

- When calculating Kt/V, where the reference value should be > 1.2, only two male patients and one female patient obtained a value lower than 1.2.

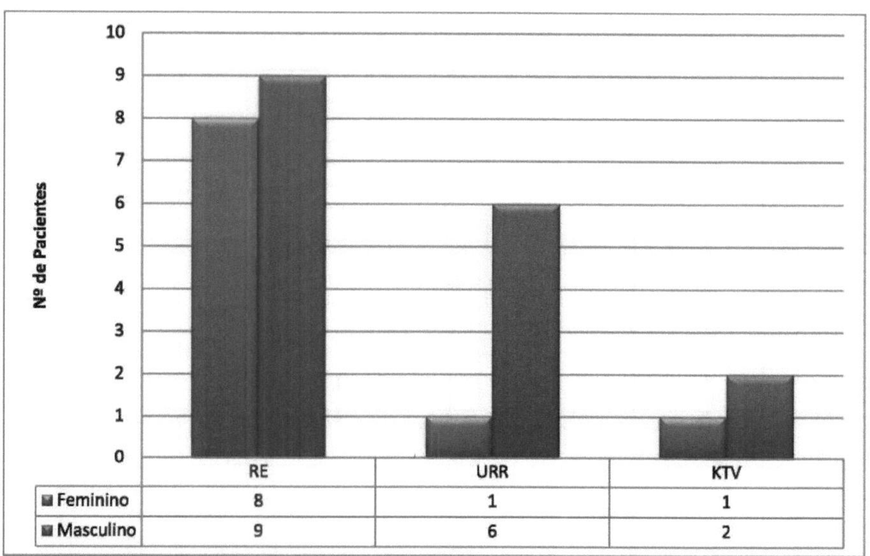

Graph 4: Distribution profile of patients with alterations in one or more of the dialysis adequacy parameters analysed in relation to gender.

Source: the author.

The data above represents only the distribution of the number of patients, selected from 29 initial patients, who presented alterations in one or more of the dialysis adequacy parameters analysed, including Recirculation (RE), Urea Reduction Rate (URR) and Kt/V. It is important to note that there was an apparent predominance of male patients for all the alterations found in the dialysis adequacy parameters analysed.

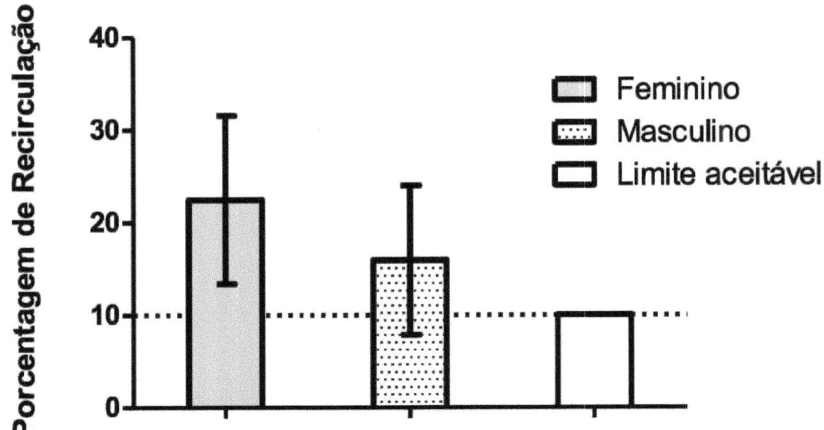

Graph 5: Influence of the gender factor on the changes found in the recirculation parameter.

Source: the author.

The data above is expressed as the mean ± standard deviation of the intermediate and high recirculation rates presented by 8 female patients (n=8) versus 9 male patients (n=9). On the Y-axis, the maximum acceptable limit was delimited (represented by the dotted line) for comparative purposes only. No significant difference was found in the analysis between the groups (t_{15} =2.49,p=0.13) (Student's t-test).

Graph five shows that the gender factor was not an important factor in determining higher rates of change in the recirculation parameter (t_{15} =2.49,p=0.13).

5.5 THE INFLUENCE OF AGE ON DIALYSIS PARAMETERS

The age factor was also analysed in detail in relation to the changes observed in the dialysis adequacy parameters stipulated in this study (Graph 6):

- Among the urea recirculation rates that characterise an intermediate or high alteration, eight patients over the age of 60 were found, compared to nine patients under the age of 60 who also showed such alterations.

- In the urea reduction rate, three patients over the age of 60 and four patients under the age of 60 had an URR of less than 65%.

- When calculating the Kt/V, two patients aged over 60 and one patient aged under 60 obtained a value of less than 1.2.

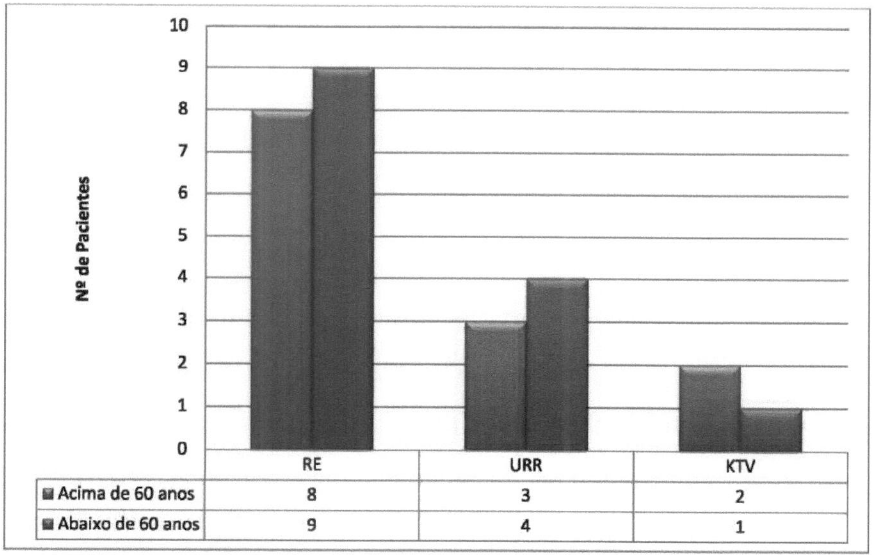

	RE	URR	KTV
Acima de 60 anos	8	3	2
Abaixo de 60 anos	9	4	1

Graph 6: Distribution profile of patients with alterations in one or more of the dialysis adequacy parameters analysed in relation to age.

Source: the author.

The data above represents only the distribution of the number of patients, selected from 29 initial patients, who showed alterations in one or more of the dialysis adequacy parameters analysed, including Recirculation (RE), Urea Reduction Rate (URR) and Kt/V. It is important to note that there was an apparent predominance of patients aged under 60 for the Recirculation and URR parameters. With regard to Kt/V, there was a predominance of patients aged over 60.

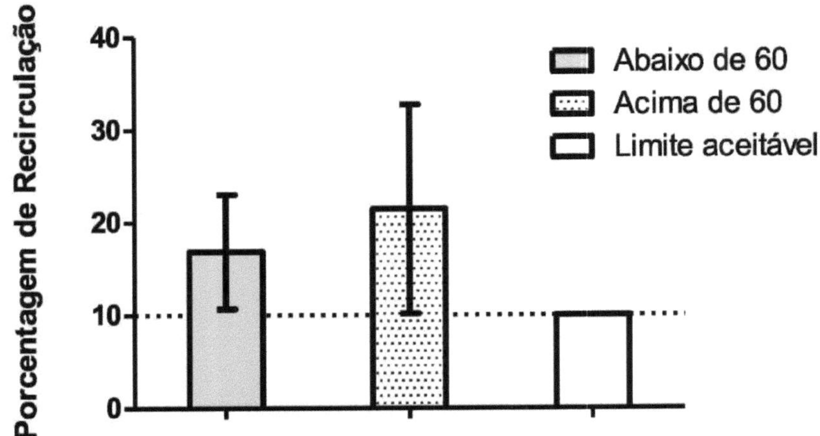

Graph 7: Influence of the age factor on the changes found in the recirculation parameter.

Source: The author.

The data was expressed as the mean ± standard deviation of the intermediate and high recirculation rate presented by 8 patients over 60 years of age (n=8) versus 9 patients under 60 years of age (n=9). On the Y-axis, the maximum acceptable limit was delimited (represented by the dotted line) for comparative purposes only. No significant difference was found in the analysis between the groups (t_{15} =1,12,p=0.30) (Student's t-test).

Analysing graph seven, it can be seen that the age factor was not significant in determining higher rates of change in recirculation (t_{15} =1,12,p=0.30).

CHAPTER 6

DISCUSSION

Dialysis is used to remove uremic fluids and waste products from the body when it is unable to remove them through renal filtration. Chronic dialysis is indicated in cases of end-stage renal disease, where uremic signs and symptoms affecting all organ systems are observed, such as nausea, vomiting, severe anorexia, mental confusion, hyperkalaemia, water overload and pericardial friction (BRUNNER; SUDDARTH et al., 2009).

Plasma urea levels should be measured monthly, and pre-dialysis values below 60 mg/dl and above 110 mg/dl are associated with an increased risk of death (DAUGIRDAS, 2000).

In an attempt to assess the efficiency of dialysis, some parameters have been proposed, which are already well described in the literature. Thus, the urea recirculation rate, the urea reduction rate and the Kt/V calculation were important parameters to indicate dialysis efficiency in the findings of this study. It is known that these parameters can be influenced by factors such as the quality of the venous access, dialysis time, dialyser and even gender and age.

6.1 QUALITY OF VENOUS ACCESS

A good venous access is one that allows adequate blood flow, without recirculation, easy puncture, aesthetically acceptable and comfortable for the client (WOLOSKER; KUZNIEC, 2007). However, in certain cases, the AVF is not of such high quality, due to the particularities of each client. It may be that this venous access has not developed as expected, characterising it as a factor that makes punctures difficult, for example.

The literature indicates a distance of 5 cm between punctures. In some cases, the patient's AVF does not allow this distance between the punctures, where the accesses are too close, causing recirculation of the arteriovenous fistula, as evidenced by excess serum urea (REIS et al, 2001).

Therefore, it is believed that the inefficiency or non-compliance with the requirements mentioned above could justify, at least in part, the changes found in the dialysis adequacy parameters (Graph 1-3).

Another important point is to assess whether the type of access used in the patients analysed in this study was really the most appropriate. This is because the results expressed here are based exclusively on the assessment of patients with AVF as the definitive access. Therefore, although the AVF is considered the best access option due to its wide range of advantages (DALLACOSTA; FIGUEIREDO, 2010), in certain cases, where the patient does not have the necessary conditions to undergo this procedure, the use of a synthetic graft such as that using PTFE (expanded polytetrafluoroethylene) may be indicated. Although it is not widely used in Brazil, it is well used in the USA and Europe, the synthetic graft has few disadvantages for the patient compared to another form of graft, which would be the use of the autogenous saphenous vein. In this case, the saphenous vein is removed from the patient's lower limb and placed in the upper limb for haemodialysis. It should be noted that the surgical procedure to remove the saphenous vein is major and can cause post-operative complications for the client, which is a major disadvantage. Through the surgical procedure in the upper limb, an end-to-side anastomosis (junction) will be formed at one end of the artery (most commonly the distal radial artery) and another end-to-side anastomosis in a vein (most commonly the basilic vein) with the graft, of sufficient length for repeated punctures. Just as the AVF has a maturation time, the graft also has a time that takes between 2 and 6 weeks to be in good condition for use, avoiding haematomas, oedema, erythema and other complications (WOLOSKER; KUZNIEC, 2007).

Another possible reason for the changes observed in dialysis parameters involves the care taken to maintain the AVF. This is because such care requires greater dedication from patients, families and health professionals, even before the fistula is made. The moment is characterised as turbulent, as the clinical condition of chronic renal failure causes the family and patient to go into crisis due to the acceptance of the disease and treatment. This is why it is important for nurses to offer support and guidance on the disease and treatment. Nurses are directly involved in patient care during haemodialysis treatment, where they are given the opportunity to plan educational interventions to enable patients and their families to care for the fistula, enabling them to understand the importance of giving greater attention and care to the treatment (MANIVA; FREITAS, 2010).

When looking at the role of nursing in relation to punctures for dialysis, one must be aware that each patient is a unique being who has a unique venous access that may also have particularities. There are cases in which the fistula is small or poorly developed, or the patient may have haematomas due to frequent punctures. In these cases, the nurse must work to find a new venous access site, trying to maintain the quality needed for dialysis to be successful (DALLACOSTA; FIGUEIREDO, 2010). Some signs and symptoms should be analysed by nurses in order to avoid complications and institute early treatment in cases of stenosis, oedema in the extremities, thrombosis, infection, bleeding and pseudoaneurysm (WOLOSKER; KUZNIEC, 2007). According to Wolosker et al. (2007, p.142) "In addition to inspection at each puncture, static and dynamic pressures and recirculation rate should be measured and calculated frequently or whenever the clinical/laboratory picture shows changes." This is how important it is for the nursing team to be prepared to act immediately and effectively to prevent and resolve haemodialysis complications in order to avoid complications and promote quality care for the client (BELTRAME et al., 2011).

Nurses must keep a close eye on their haemodialysis clients, as patients with kidney disorders have hydroelectrolytic imbalances and need to be assessed continuously to detect possible problems such as fluid retention. One way of controlling this *is to* record fluid intake and output, which documents water parameters, taking into account the amount of fluid ingested orally or parenterally, and the volume of water excreted, including urine, vomit, sweating and diarrhoea. Another important parameter is the patient's weight, indicating the patient's need for water and defining signs of fluid overload or deficit. When assessing a client whose fluid intake exceeds the kidneys' capacity to excrete this fluid, we say that they are fluid overloaded and may present weight gain, oedema, rales, shortness of breath, decreased urea, low haematocrit, among others. In the case of inadequate intake, this organism is said to be volume depleted due to a deficit in fluid volume and may show signs and symptoms such as weight loss, decreased skin turgour, high haematocrit, increased urea level, among others

(BRUNNER; SUDDARTH et al., 2009).

According to Dallacosta and Figueiredo (2010, p. 7) "It is important to emphasise that maintaining vascular access is an essential activity of haemodialysis nurses and that good recirculation results reflect the work of nursing". In other words, the nurse's tool is care, and this care will reflect on the best quality of dialysis and the patient's quality of life.

6.2 DIALYSIS TIME

With regard to dialysis time, using a high blood flow velocity, a dialyser with high-flow membranes and a short dialysis session can cause good urea removal, but will not always guarantee satisfactory clearance of substances with a higher molecular weight. Some HD centres advocate a long, slow approach to the procedure. In these centres, a low to medium flow dialyser is used, the speed of blood flow is lower and the duration of dialysis is 4 hours or more. The aim is to ensure that the Kt/V has a value > 1.0. It is not known whether a longer dialysis session is beneficial or not, there are many controversies (DAUGIRDAS, 2008).

One hypothesis that could indicate the inefficiency of dialysis in this study correlates with the time (hours) or frequency (times per week) of this procedure for each patient. The Kt/V parameter uses dialysis time in its formula, hence the influence of this factor as one of the reasons for the altered Kt/V indices shown in graph 3. One option is to rethink the time and/or frequency of patients receiving intermediate and/or high recirculation as an alternative for dialysis efficiency.

6.3 DIALISATOR

The dialyser is a tube with four inlets, two of which communicate with a blood compartment and the other two with a dialysis compartment. In the hollow fibre dialyser (also called a capillary), which is the material used in the clinic researched, the blood flows into a chamber at the top end of the cylindrical compartment, following thousands of small capillaries grouped into a bundle. The blood passes through these fibres and the dialysis solution, undergoing the purification of solutes. After passing through the capillaries, the blood is collected in a chamber at the lower end of the cylindrical compartment, and is then returned to the patient (STONE, 2008).

Therefore, the dialyser is known as an artificial kidney, which serves as a synthetic semi-permeable membrane, replacing the glomeruli and renal tubules as a filter for the compromised kidneys. Diffusion is the removal of toxins and waste products from the blood, which move from the area of highest concentration to the area of lowest concentration, the dialysate in this case. Dialysate is a solution that contains important electrolytes in ideal extracellular concentrations. The level of electrolytes in the client's blood can be controlled via the dialysate bath. The semi-permeable membrane prevents larger cells such as erythrocytes and proteins from diffusing. Another important objective of HD is the removal of excess fluids, in which water is removed from the blood through osmosis, where the water moves from the medium of higher concentration to an area of lower concentration. In the ultrafiltration method, which is the most widely used, water is removed from the higher pressure medium to the lower pressure medium. We mustn't forget the body's buffer system, which is maintained using a dialysate bath loaded with bicarbonate or acetate. Heparin is also administered to prevent blood clotting in the dialysis circuit (BRUNNER;

SUDDARTH et al., 2009).

With regard to dialyser size, this should be geared to the size of the patient. Therefore, we can associate the high recirculation rate in the accesses of the subjects used in this research with the inadequate dialyser size, in which small patients can use smaller dialysers (e.g. 17), and more obese patients use larger dialysers (e.g. 21). Dialysers with a large surface area generally have high urea clearance. If an obese, tall patient is using a small dialyser (with a small surface area) they may experience inefficient dialysis due to low urea clearance.

6.4 GENDER INFLUENCE

Regarding the influence of the gender factor on the alterations found, there was a predominance of males for all the alterations found in the dialysis efficiency parameters analysed. This corroborates data from the 2009 Brazilian Dialysis Census, in which 57% of patients undergoing treatment were male (SESSO, 2010). This finding can be interpreted from different perspectives, which the genders show in relation to self-care both in the pre-pathological condition and in the face of dialysis. For example, males show less self-care and, consequently, less demand for health professionals, in contrast to the results obtained for females (COSTA, 2003). This behavioural difference may be related to cultural factors, where men learn to think and act without caring about their health (NOVAES et al., 2009), since this is culturally considered a sign of weakness for men (COSTA, 2003).

It is therefore a challenge for nursing professionals to realise how cultural factors may be influencing the quality of patients' health and thus find the best way to educate patients in the face of this cultural barrier.

6.5 THE INFLUENCE OF AGE

Over the years, from adulthood onwards, the functional capacity of each system that makes up an individual's body is reduced due to the natural and physiological process of ageing (KUSUMOTA; OLIVEIRA; MARQUES, 2009). With advancing age, the kidney undergoes structural and functional changes, such as a significant decrease in renal mass (reduction in the size of the organ) and a reduction in the number of functional nephrons (ROSNER, 2009). Under normal conditions, these renal alterations can be functionally compensated for by adaptations in renal haemodynamics, but under pathological conditions, the kidney saturates its compensatory capacity, which results in greater chances of the individual developing clinically relevant damage (ROSNER, 2009). For example, a higher incidence of acute renal failure has been associated with older patients (ABDEL-KADER; PALEVSKY, 2009). In addition, there has been a growing increase in the number of elderly people with chronic kidney disease (CKD) (KUSUMOTA; OLIVEIRA; MARQUES, 2009).

According to the information mentioned above, the expected findings of this study would be that there would be a greater number of elderly patients on haemodialysis and, even more so, that these patients would show greater alterations in the parameters related to dialysis efficiency when compared to other patients under 60 years of age. However, under the conditions stipulated in this study, the age factor did not seem to be important. One possible justification could be that although age is one of the main risk factors, it is only one of several risk factors associated with the development of renal system diseases. Therefore, obesity, hypertension, diabetes, autoimmune diseases, neoplasms, systemic infections, family history of kidney disease (VASSALOTTI; FOX; BECKER, 2010), as well as the use of drugs of abuse (PANTELIAS; GRAPSA, 2011), which is closely associated with young adults, are important factors that contribute to the onset of kidney disease.

What can be concluded is that kidney disease associated with the need for dialysis often seems to depend on a combination of genetic and environmental factors. The great challenge for nursing is to identify kidney disease (and other pathologies in general) earlier (since kidney disease rarely causes symptoms), with the aim of promoting and preventing the health/disease process. However, nurses face the challenge of educating patients and their families about palliative care methods in order to carry out treatment and rehabilitation in this process. Although for the findings of this study the age factor did not prove to be important for the alterations found, attention to this factor will be increasing, since according to the analysis of demographic variables in Brazil there will be an increase in the longevity of the population throughout 2030, towards an increasingly aged age pattern (IBGE, 2006).

CHAPTER 7

CONCLUSION

The Dialysis Adequacy parameters again proved to be important tools for controlling this procedure, since they were able to detect the inefficiency and efficiency of the dialysis procedure. In this way, it becomes possible for the nursing professional to investigate the source and the appropriate intervention to resolve the problem. In addition, it is clear that it is important to observe parameters for adjustment on a monthly basis, since serum urea above acceptable levels can lead to an increase in patient morbidity and mortality.As a final contribution, it is believed that from this research the nursing team will be able to look for ways of carrying out haemodialysis, with a view to improving its quality. Nurses have a unique role to play in controlling dialysis. They can use the parameters mentioned in this research and also pay attention to the signs and symptoms that the patient presents. It is also the nurse's duty to encourage self-care on the part of patients and their families and/or carers, who should follow the guidelines on diet, maintenance of the AVF, and other care that will have a direct effect on the efficiency of dialysis and a better quality of life.Therefore, the importance of nurses in haemodialysis should be clear, as they are competent and play a major role in the care and prevention of health problems for their clients.

REFERENCES

ABDEL-KADER, K.; PALEVSKY, P. Acute Kidney Injury in the Elderly. **Clin. Geriatr. Med.** 2009 August; 25(3): 331-358. Available at: <http://www.ncbi.nlm.nih.gov/pmc/articles/PMC2748997/pdf/nihmsll3646.pdf>. Accessed on: 20 October 2014.

AKISKAL et al. **Merk Manual:** health for the family. Peritoneal dialysis. Oceano Grupo Editorial.

2009. Available at: <http://www.manuahnerck.net/?id=149&cn=2106>. Accessed on: 20 October 2014.

ANTCZAK, S. E. et al. **Basic physiopathology.** Translation by Ana Karine Ramos Brum. Rio de Janeiro: Guanabara Koogan, 2005.

BELTRAME, V. et al. Nursing interventions in haemodialysis treatment complications. **Ágora: R. Divulg. Cient.,** ISSN 2237-9010, Mafra, v. 18, n. 1, 2011. Available at: < http://www.periodicos.unc.br/index.php/agora/article/view/252/334>. Accessed on: 29 August 2014.

BRUNNER, L. S.; SUDDARTH, D. S.; SMELTZER, S. C.; BARE, B.; HINKLE, J. L.; CHEEVER, K. H. G. **Treatise on medical-surgical nursing.** 11th ed. Rio de Janeiro: Guanabara Koogan, 2009, volume 3.

CABRAL, LC; TRINDADE, F.R.; BRANCO, F.M.F.C.; BALDOINO, L.S.; SILVA, M.L.R.; LAGO, E.C. The perception of haemodialysis patients regarding the arteriovenous fistula. **R. Interd.** 2013 Apr-Jun; 6(2):15-25. Available at: < http://revistainterdisciplinar.uninovafapi.edu.br/index.php/revinter/article/view/43/pdf_44>. Accessed on: 05 October 2014.

COSTA, R. G. Health and masculinity: reflections from a gender perspective. **Brazilian Journal of Population Studies.** V.20, n.l, jan./jun. 2003. Available at: < http://www.abep.nepo.unicamp.br/docs/rev_inf/vol20_nl_2003/vol20_nl_2003_7artigo_p79 a92.pdf>. Accessed on: 20 October 2014.

DALLACOSTA, F.M.; FIGUEIREDO, A. E. P. L. **Recirculation in the vascular access of haemodialysis patients.** Rio Grande do Sul, 9 pg. 2010.

DAUGIRDAS, J. T. Prescription of Chronic Haemodialysis: An Approach to Urea Kinetics. In: DAUGIRDAS, J. T.; BLAKE, Peter G.; ING, T. S. **Manual of dialysis.** Editora Guanabara, 4° ed. 2008. Chap. 06. Available at: < https://www.bibliomed.com.br/bibliomed/bmbooks/nefrolog/livrol/cap/cap06.htm>. Accessed on: 01 October 2014.

DAUGIRDAS, J. T. Second Generation Logarithmic Estimates of Single-Pool Variable Volume Kt/V: an Analysis Error. **J. Am. Soc. Nephrol.** 4: 1205-13,1993. Available at: <http://jasn.asnjoumals.org/content/4/5/1205.full.pdf?origin=publication_detail>. Accessed on: 19 October 2014

DIEPENBROCK, N. H. **Intensive care.** Technical review by Denise de Assis Corrêa Sória. Rio de Janeiro: Guanabara Koogan, 2005.

DRAIBE, S. A.; CENDOROGLO, M.; NADALETTO, M. A. Update on dialysis: Adequacy in chronic haemodialysis. **J. Bras. Nefrol.** 2000. Available at: < http://www.jbn.org.br/detalhe_artigo.asp?id=574>. Accessed on: 16 October 2014.

IBGE - Brazilian Institute of Geography and Statistics. **Sociodemographic Indicators:** Prospective for Brazil 1991-2030 - São Paulo. Rio de Janeiro, 2006. Available at: < http://www.ibge.gov.br/home/estatistica/populacao/projecao_da_populacao/publicacao_UNF

PA.pdf>. Accessed on: 18 October 2014.

KDOQI. **Clinical Practice Guidelines For Haemodialysis Adequacy.** National Kidney Foundation, Inc, 2006. Available at: <http://www2.kidney.org/professionals/KDOQI/guideline_upHD_PD_VA/hd_guide2.htm>. Accessed on: 05 October 2014.

KOEPE, G. B. O.; ARAÚJO, S. T. C. The perception of haemodialysis clients regarding the arteriovenous fistula in their bodies. **Acta Paulista de Enfermagem,** São Paulo, v. 21, n. supplement, p. 147-51, 2008. Available at: <http://www.scielo.br/scielo.php?script=sci_arttext&pid=S0103-21002008000500002>. Accessed on: 29 September 2014.

KUSUMOTA, L.; OLIVEIRA, M. P.; MARQUES S. The elderly on dialysis. **Acta Paul. Enfermagem.** 2009; 22:546-50. Available at: < http://www.scielo.br/scielo.php?script=sci_arttext&pid=S0103-21002009000800020>. Accessed on: 19 October 2014.

MANIVA, S.J.C.F.; FREITAS, C.H.A. The haemodialysis patient: self-care with the arteriovenous fistula. **Rev. Rene. Fortaleza,** v. 11, n. 1, p. 152-160, jan./mar.2010. Available at: http://www.revistarene.ufc.br/revista/index.php/revista/article/view/358/pdf>. Accessed on: 10 October 2014.

Nefroclínica Dialysis Manual - updated March 2011. Available at: < http://www.nefroclinica.com/paginas/manual_rotinas.pdf>. Accessed on: 17 August 2014.

Dialysis Manual/Nephrology Department of the Getúlio Vargas Hospital. Updated March 2012. 80 pg. Available at: <http://www.hgv.pi.gov.br/download/201204/HGV25_43447dbcff.pdf>. Accessed on: 17 August 2014.

MORTON, P. G. et al. **Critical care nursing:** a holistic approach. 8. ed. Rio de Janeiro: Guanabara Koogan, 2007. 1389 p.

NOVAES, N. B. et al. Self-care: a gender issue? **Rev. Enferm. Herediana.** 2009;2(2):73-79. Available at: < http://www.upch.edu.pe/faenf/images/stories/articulorevista2_2/genero_2_2_4>. Accessed on: 21 October 2014.

PANTELIAS, K.; GRAPSA, E. Drug abuse and Kidney. **Hippokratia Medicai Journal,** 2011, 15 (Suppl 2): 4-8. Available at: <http://hippokratia.gr/images/PDF/15Sup2/831.pdf>. Accessed on: 18 October 2014.

REIS, E.M.K. et al. Percentage of blood recirculation in different forms of needle insertions in arteriovenous fistulas of patients undergoing haemodialysis treatment. **Rev. Esc. Enf. USP,** v.35, n. 1, p. 41-5, mar. 2001. Available at: < http://www.revistas.usp.br/reeusp/article/viewFile/41192/44740>. Accessed on: 06 September 2014.

ROSNER, M. H. Acute Kidney Injury in the Elderly. **ASN (American Society of Nephrology) Geriatrics Nephrology Online Curriculum, p. 1-6,2009.**

Available at: <https://www.asn-online.org/education/distanceleaming/curricula/geriatrics/Chapterl8.pdf>. Accessed on: 20 October 2014.

SESSO, R. C. C. et al. Brazilian Dialysis Census, 2009. **J. Bras. Nefrol.,** v 32, n. 4, 2010. Available at: <http://www.scielo.br/scielo.php?pid=S0101-28002010000400007&script=sci_arttext>. Accessed on: 16 October 2014.

SHINABERGER, J. H. Quantitation of Dialysis: Historical Perspective. **Rev. Semin. Dial.** Pg. 238 to 245. 2001. Disponível em: <http://onlinelibrary.wiley.eom/doi/10.1046/j.1525-139X.2001.00063.x/abstract;jsessionid=855564FlB69001B6B8AE482E84336264.f03t03>. Accessed on: 21 August 2014.

STONE, J. C. V. Haemodialysis apparatus. In: DAUGIRDAS, J. T.; BLAKE, Peter G.; ING, T. S. **Manual of dialysis.** Editora Guanabara, 4° ed. 2008. Chap. 03. Available at: < http://www.bibliomed.com.br/bibliomed/bmbooks/nefrolog/livrol/cap/cap03.htm>. Accessed on: 01 October 2014.

VASSALOTTI, J. A.; FOX, C. H.; BECKER, B. N. Risk factors and screening for chronic kidney disease. **Adv. Chronic. Kidney. Dis.** 2010 May;17(3):237-45. Available at: < http://www.ncbi.nlm.nih.gov/pubmed/20439092>. Accessed on: 20 October 2014.

WOLOSKER, N.; KUZNIEC, S. **Vascular accesses for chemotherapy and haemodialysis.** São Paulo, SP: Atheneu, 2007. 166 p.

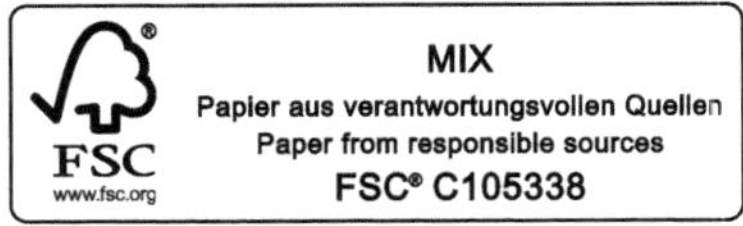

Printed by Books on Demand GmbH, Norderstedt / Germany